7 VALUABLE TIPS TO BEING AN OUTSTANDING PHYSICAL, OCCUPATIONAL & SPEECH THERAPIST

The 7 Gems That Set You Apart from the Rest

Dr. Michael T. Maghari

PT, DPT, CES, CPAHA

Copyright © Dr. Michael T. Maghari, 2018

Disclaimer

The information in this book is to be used for informational and educational purposes only. The author will not account in any way for any results that stem from the use of the contents herein. While conscious and creative attempts have been made to ensure that all information provided herein is as accurate and useful as possible, the author is not legally bound to be responsible for any damage caused by the accuracy as well as use/misuse of this information.

Dedication

I dedicate this book to my family (my Mom who recently passed away and to my hard-working Dad), relatives, friends, patients, colleagues and people I met who are still living and have gone ahead.

Acknowledgement

I acknowledge that apart from the Grace and Wisdom of GOD, I wouldn't be able to come up with this book. I give all The Glory and Honor to GOD!

Author's Note

I was inspired to write this book to help therapists achieve their true potential by applying the principles found in this book. My greatest wish is that as you read and put into use these tips, they will be of immense help to you.

To GOD be The Glory!

~Dr. Michael T. Maghari

Table of Contents

Introduction

As one of the inevitable requirements of the twenty-first century, there's a dramatic change in the social, religious and moral lifestyles of people. Most of the essentials of contemporary life demand these changes. And as many people are getting involved in change in paradigm, they are in need of confidence, efficacy, and esteem in themselves than never before. Every field of human endeavor requires those in need to possess of one skill or unique individual traits in order to respond successfully to its demands.

Specific skills assist professionals in dealing with the challenges of the workplace and certain practices. These skills range from the cognitive, psychological, social and so on. These are made combinative to become effective and to enable the individual not only to solve problems using informed methods but also to do so more creatively, critically and with the desired compassion. These skills requirements are not dissimilar from those in the field of therapy.

Daily, people face physical, psychological, mental issues and stress in life. Some of them are prone to weakness, low self-esteem, anger and self-harm. For them, to adapt and be flexible every day, they need professionals who are trained to attend to them and see that they have a more fulfilling life. These, amongst many others, are the goals of a therapist. Before I give you the 7 Ps or life gems to be an outstanding therapist, below is a summary of the three dimensions of therapy disciplines we are all aware of.

Physical Therapy

Physical therapists are health care professionals that treat individuals of different ages and lifespan, from a newborn baby to the oldest individual who have health related and medical problems restricting their mobility and performance of daily activities and functions.

Physical Therapists examines the patient, develop a plan of care then provides treatment using therapeutic exercises, manual skills, use of physical agents and modalities and neuromuscular techniques and interventions to restore function, reduce pain, promote movement and the prevention of injury or disability.

Physical Therapists practices in a broad range of clinical settings from nursing homes, hospitals, outpatient clinics, schools, home health agencies, sports and fitness facilities and corporate work settings.

Physical Therapists requires a license to practice in the state or states they intend to work.

Occupational Therapy

Occupational Therapists are health care professionals that help individuals from different lifespan across the continuum of care in restoration of function through the therapeutic use of daily activities or occupations.

The treatment includes helping children with disabilities to participate fully in schools and social functions, help individuals recover lost functions and regain skills resulting from an injury, illness or disability.

Occupational Therapists practices in a broad range of clinical settings from nursing homes, hospitals, outpatient clinics, schools, home health agencies and corporate work settings.

Occupational Therapists requires a license to practice in the state or states they intend to work.

Speech Therapy

Speech Therapists or speech language pathologists are healthcare professionals that work with people who have problems or difficulty with their speech, language, thinking and swallowing.

They perform assessment, diagnosis and treatment of speech, language, social and cognitive communications and swallowing disorders in both children and adults. They also work in the prevention of conditions mentioned above.

Speech therapists practices in a broad range of clinical settings from nursing homes, hospitals, outpatient clinics, schools and home health agencies.

Speech language pathologists requires a license to practice in the state or states they intend to work.

The 7 Gems That Set You Apart as a Therapist

Having given a summary of the three dimensions of therapy disciplines in the healthcare and medical field, the 7 Ps to be discussed include patience, passion, purpose, persistence, principles, proactive and praise.

Patience

Many things contribute to the success of therapy and how long it may take. Our patients are individuals, and each has his/her own unique time of responding to therapy treatments and sessions. It is a rapid and clear-cut experience for some people while others find it slow and tedious to react accordingly.

As a therapist, we should be patient enough to create a relationship and interaction between us and our clients. This is for no other reason than to have a working environment for us and to boost the confidence of our patients. we need to make them realize that they are not passing through this road alone, but, instead, we are with them, supporting and helping them to the end. let our patience serve as a virtue worthy of influencing them to understand how hard we're trying to see that you both achieve the desired result.

We need patience and time to work with family members and to get their full participation. our task as a therapist is not only to our patients at this time but also to the patient's families, by taking the time to create the awareness that you cannot achieve this without them.

Some cases are more complex and rigorous than others. we need patience to deal with all of them whether we are physical, occupational or speech therapists.

The moment we run out of patience and decide to reduce the number of days we attend to our clients, there is a quick relapse our patients are made to suffer. Thus, we are not expected to cancel appointments but to keep our work, be patient, and make it worth your passion. If we do this, we do not only stand out as therapists but also encourage a positive impact on our clients and fast-track a maximum recovery process. If we really love our career as a therapist, patience is one of the greatest tools we need to have. we will be patient enough to be with our clients during their recovery process. A good example of patience is from the Bible, where Jacob, whose loved Rachel so much that he had to wait another seven years for her. Notice what the Bible says concerning this:

As a therapist, our love for our profession and for our patients is enough to carry us through all the challenges that may surface with time.

Let us try to always keep our appointments even when there are circumstances that may warrant us or not. The need for keeping appointments is not only expected of the patient, but also for the therapist. hold yourself accountable as a therapist. Once we are with our patients, we should be patient enough to eliminate all possible distractions both within and without, to create the necessary environment for concentration, connection and improved relationship with our patients.

Take time to have a teachable heart and always open for new learning and study various methods of implementing new findings and therapy techniques that are sure to be beneficial to our patients. Exercise patience in assuring them that they will be okay as they trust us their therapist. Remember, therapy involves participation, effort, alertness, concentration and a behavioral or mindset change, all of which takes time to attain.

As a therapist, let us encourage our patients to practice on their own and carry over the exercises we taught them. This is where the home exercise program and patient education are valuable and are very helpful to patients and clients.

Therapists practice and exhibits patience on a daily basis. It is a career where service is at the forefront of what we offer and do. Be patient! It is one of the precious life gems that will make us stand out and be unique in the efforts and service we show to the profession.

Passion

If you were to mention what you love doing so well, then it is certain that you are very passionate about that thing. Since it is what you love doing, it means you seldom grow tired of doing it. It is like an energy to your soul and body, and it makes you feel good. Passion is a gem we can't do without.

The definition of passion as it is given in this book is simply *"loving what you do and doing what you love."* So, from this definition, we can see that there is the active work of a positive emotion there, and that is love. You can take a cue of understanding from the love between two people. The sight is a good thing to behold. When there is love for someone or a thing, there is a bond of oneness and unity.

This means that passion has its drive from the inward part of a person. Passion provides energy. It is like a fire that burns and consumes us above all other things set aside. When you see someone that has passion for what he/she does, such person does work with a difference.

The importance of passion as a life gem is so that we can make a difference wherever we are and wherever we go now in our therapy journey.

As a therapist, the need for passion in our practice cannot be over-emphasized. Passion, that unquenchable zeal for loving what you do and doing what you love, equips us with the energy and fire to give more of ourselves to our patients, their families and people around us. In life, generally, the lack of zeal for a course does not guarantee a successful outcome. This also goes for therapy. Be in tune with your driving force.

There's nothing that should give us happiness and fulfillment other than the fact that we wake up and realize that we are therapists and are blessed to be one. Be driven by that passion that you are making a big impact and that you are changing the world by helping others. Let's always remember our passion.

Persistence

There is a saying "against all odds"? Well, this is what persistence is all about. It is your ability to keep pushing on, despite all the challenges that are not in your favor.

Persistence simply means, *"never giving up."* It is one of the secrets to a fruitful and fulfilling life. Persistence has its strength in the fact that things are possible.

Being persistent is like a spring of water that is ever flowing and never ceases. Its glory lies in continuity.

To be a therapist, we need to be relentless and determined in achieving the goals we have set for ourselves and for our patients. I always advise people that to have great results they need to be consistent and continue at their endeavor. This is very important, especially if we are to deliver the care and intervention our patient needs.

Determination is what drives any venture or endeavor into becoming a success. Once you have started a session with a patient, do not allow any other factor to discourage you or lead you into giving up. While you may enjoy and even love your sessions with some patients, others always test your tenacity. But do not forget that although you are there as an expert, it is the patient who exercises the prerogative of responding to, and getting better after, treatment. You serve as a professional and trained guardian in the recovery process.

As a therapist, I advise you always persist even when things do not seem to go according to your plans. Let's not give up on our patients. Don't give up on yourself as a therapist.

Through persistence, you can break any barrier, win any war and climb any mountain. Persistence is one of the mottos of a champion.

Do you want to be a champion? If yes, then, persist in that area that you have recorded failure, and continue to aim for success.

The fact that you have failed initially is a sign that there is something good that is within your reach that you are about to get if only you put in the necessary effort and be persistent.

Look up! there is a bright light ahead in
the dark tunnel!

Purpose

One of the most important questions we need to ask ourselves in life is this: "What is my purpose in life?" This six-worded question, as simple and straight as it sounds, is the singular force that has redirected the steps of many people who have become great today. I want you to look at the details of your life and ponder: What is the reason behind your every action? To what extent, and how, do you fit in the bigger scheme of life? These questions will go a long way to help us discover our true purpose in life. Because without purpose, our life and all its goals will not only lack a plan but, also an establishment. Our dreams and ambitions need clarity of vision.

How can we serve God through other people when we have no idea of our purpose in life? Seems impossible. So, also in our field as therapists.

Purpose is one of the essential gems to make us stand out as therapists. It is what gives meaning to our practice, and without it, it is hard to become positive and exercise the other gems presented here. A clearly stated purpose will not only give direction but also help to make the changes necessary in coping during crises. Purpose helps to renew our energy for growth and learning new things in our field, teaching us how to be receptive to the essential aspects of our well-being not only as a therapist but also as an individual who also needs compassion and time.

Once we have identified our purpose as therapists, it can help as a constant reminder of our values, beliefs, needs, and goals. It will make us readily available to learn new techniques, tools, and dream-works throughout our careers.

Therapists who have identified their purpose in their profession can handle the emotional problems or stressors that come with the job. Most of the life-altering occurrences mildly affect them. In the sense that, having studied various problems in their patients, they also apply the many lessons to their own lives. This is not to say that therapists are immune to these anomalies. What this implies, in essence, is that their effect is minimal.

So, let us be in tune and in line with our purpose.

Job in the Bible knew this when he said:

"I know that you can do all things and that no purpose of yours can be thwarted"

~ Job 42:2, ESV

Reminder: Know your purpose as a therapist and follow it with all your heart and mind. Even George Washington, the first President of the United States of America, advises the same: "Make sure you are doing what God wants you to do--then do it with all your strength."

You will be different and will make a difference!

As you know your Purpose in life, you
will know your destination!

Proactive

Being proactive in life means you have to be ready to standup to the task and do things ahead of time. It means you should have a good perception and a plan of action. It is you sensing that situations are getting bad and rising to take control of them before they get out of hands. Being proactive as a therapist requires us to observe and do the following:

1. ***Think ahead***– this will help us better in our field or profession. we go out of our way to learn from those who have gone ahead of us, those who are visionaries, trailblazers and dream catchers that have made an impact in the profession and learn as much as we can from them. The essence of this

is to make you ready for challenges, have more available time, and be strong enough to play the desired role in our patient's life. Remember as soon as someone requires our services as therapists; it means they are ready to share their life with us from that moment until we feel they are independent enough to face life and its challenges ahead of them. So, be proactive enough to think ahead and find even betters way for them to have a better life.

2. ***Set short term and long-term goals for yourself and your patients*** – we do this all the time in our practice as therapists. This means we are able to foresee outcomes in our client's case that are not visible in the present. You

have a clear-cut presentation on how they might be able to aim for, and live, a healthier and happier life. our submissions should be decisive enough to foster a change in their attitude, even if they are not responding to sessions as we must have hoped they would. Let us remember, we don't give up on them. Some of them might be people who have either given up on themselves or are on the verge of doing so. Do not give up on them. Set goals for them that envision them capable of living a full and active lifestyle in whatever situation and station in life they are in.

3. ***Remain interested and positive with your patients***. They will adopt

this attitude with you in a way you do not expect. They may not attain the heights you would want them to immediately, but if they have an idea that you believe they can, and they should, you are in for a big surprise. This is influential if we need to make ourselves stand out as therapists. Be proactively positive in your dealings with your patients, each and every session. People of all ages want to be loved, understood, cherished and respected. As our patients share their social and personal life with us, appreciate them for doing so; cherish the secrets they have shared with you. Love them for doing so, listen to them, understand and communicate with them the great joys that shows

you are there to make them move
ahead and make a difference in their
lives, their families and people around
them.

Principles

"For the Lord gives wisdom; from his mouth come knowledge and understanding; he stores up sound wisdom for the upright; he is a shield to those who walk in integrity, guarding the paths of justice and watching over the way of his saints."

~ Proverbs 2:6-8 ESV

The place we stand in life is our principles. It is the place where our integrity is tested and weighed. Principles help us possess discipline in our beliefs and equip us with the necessary tools to make our tasks achievable.

As therapists, we are expected to have principles guiding us in our practice. If we have principles that we are entirely in tune with and are consistently faithful, it will be evident to others and for us to lead by example.

There are principles of therapy that we need to know and imbibe into our practice, and at each stage of our career. Our professional boards and the organizations in our respective disciplines that we represent (Physical, Occupational and Speech) have set rules and guidelines for the safe practice and good moral conduct for us to abide and follow.

On a personal basis, it becomes imperative to set a model of integrity, honesty and discipline as part of our guiding principles.

One of the essence of principles in therapy is to build trust between us and our patients, starting at the beginning of each session, before the challenges begins, then to be carried over after the end of each treatment sessions and after discharge of patients in the program.

It will consolidate us in our patient's eyes as the professional we are meant to be, and a principled therapist is more likely to be more helpful and efficient in their overall plan of care.

"Do no harm to your patients, going an extra mile of service and make them feel that you genuinely care for their health and wellbeing are good principles to live by in our practice as therapist."

We might have come across patients who show greater vulnerability that put our character to the test. But as a principled man or woman, our connection to our patients should be beneficial, assuring, trustworthy and will produce good results.

Integrity is crucial to us as a person. It is the summation of our character and gives us out as someone to be trusted.

Let people know you, to be steadfast in your belief and what you stand for in life as a man and woman of integrity. It is the path for us to follow in our practice as a therapist.

One of my favorite examples of integrity, honesty, and discipline is Daniel in the

Bible. He is the prophet of God in his time.

Daniel's strong moral principles of conviction and virtue enabled him to influence three other youths in captivity: Hananiah, Mishael, and Azariah (Shadrach, Meshach, and Abednego) who refused to bow down to the Golden Image of king Nebuchadnezzar of Babylon. Daniel's choice to live with integrity had prevented him earlier in life from defiling himself with the royal food. What was Daniel's reward? The Bible reported: *"And God gave Daniel favor and compassion in the sight of the chief of the eunuchs"* (Daniel 1:9, ESV). Soon, it didn't take long for Daniel's disciplined life and integrity to be noticed by the king, who elevated him above his peers.

Daniel was a man committed to God, who refused to compromise even in the midst of danger, right into the lion's den! And God did not forsake him.

Be forewarned by the words of the Apostle James that reflects doublemindedness:

To sum it all up, I will leave you with these sayings and a statement regarding Principles that we could all benefit from:

"To have the principles of skills and competency is good and important but to add integrity and good character is best."

"Strive and make it a priority to be a person of Integrity and honesty and you will be a person whom people can trust."

"The principles of Integrity and good character coupled with competency and efficiency sets you apart from the rest and will give you good standing to your patients, their families, colleagues and every people you get in contact with on a regular basis."

Praise

Everyone desires praise in life. Imagine going through life without a single person ever stopping you on the road or in the middle of a task to tell you how appreciative they are of the work you have done for them or are doing for them. We all want to be appreciated for the little efforts we put into doing a task. Even to live in spite of hard circumstances and difficulty is not an easy thing. Let us give praise to our patients for struggling to live against the odds posed by their challenges. Let them know how happy you are with their progress, whether big or small. Praise them for their improvement and recovery.

Giving praise is important because it's a form of encouragement that helps to motivate our patients to achieve their treatment goals. When we give praise or encouragement, it should be at the right place and at the right time.

Praise, especially positive praise, in therapy is an effective means of encouraging our patients. Once you've noticed something is wrong with your patient, or he or she is not responding to sessions as they used to, our duty is to encourage them by telling them how much wonderfully they have been doing before and how much more capable they can be if they put more effort and energy.

In my experience working as a physical therapist, my patients and colleagues would joke and call me or say to me "very good!" because that's the word I used a lot to motivate my patients in their therapy sessions.

Look for the positive things in your patients and tell them how they are doing well. Be genuine about this. They are our patients, they can see through us as much as we can see through them. Be honest in your praise. Appreciate them and the other qualities or attitudes they have that you think are worth praising.

When after a session you have given your patient a test to do, and he or she does it well, let them know how excited you are about it. Go over it and provide them with feedback, tell them what you think they have done that makes it great. What improvement have they made that's making you excited. By praising your patients, you are upping their belief in themselves. Their self-esteem is raised, and they will be more motivated to work with you in every therapy session.

Let them know that each attempt that they continually make means they are showing signs of significant improvement. Even a thing as showing up early to a session is an attempt that needs to be praised. Let them know how you appreciate this, and it might go a long way in their recovery.

Don't hold back the praises. Let us use them as often as they are needed. Everyone loves to be praised and complimented. We always want to have a sense of accomplishing something all by ourselves. Et us use this strategy to ensure that there are positive reinforcements in each session between us and our patients. praise is a stimulus that will encourage future cooperation between us and our patients.

Praise helps to contribute to our success as therapists, whether in the field of physical, occupational or speech therapy.

In essence, take this gem as one of the essential tools to help patients and clients recover; a simple praise will go a long way in therapy!

Conclusion

As stated at the beginning, the twenty-first-century demands more from humans than ever before. At work, in schools, homes, hospitals, etc. people constantly have physical, psychological, and total breakdown, increasing the demand for our services as a therapist demands. As an occupational, physical and speech therapist, we will find a lot of challenges and competition in the healthcare field. This should neither deter nor discourage us. Instead, we should train ourselves to be more patient, passionate, persistent, purposeful, proactive, principled, and free with praise to deliver the best healthcare services our patient needs and deserves. My hope is that this book will serve as a valuable resource and inspirational guide in the practice of physical, occupational and speech therapy services that will impact the delivery of healthcare in this country and around the world.

I wish all of us Success! To GOD be The Glory!

9 781728 770048